Waiting for Dad

A Yoga Story for Kids

Written and Illustrated by Lakshmi Gosyne

Congratulations on being a giveaway winner!

Lakshmi Gosyne

Nov. 2013.

ISBN-13: 978-1480273252

ISBN-10: 1480273252

Photo Credits
Copyright © 2012 by Jaya and Ravi Maharajh photographing images of Arjun and Ashvin

Illustrations
Copyright © 2012 by Lakshmi Gosyne with the following exceptions:
Tiger Image from http://www.flickr.com/photos/binderdonedat/2702587619/
Earth and Moon Images from NASA http://www.nasa.gov
Briefcase drawings based on Baratani black briefcase

The intent of this book is to introduce yoga to young children through story in a fun engaging way. The author does not take responsibility or liability for the improper replication of yoga poses while reading this book. Please exercise caution and discretion when stretching, breathing, and modelling the yoga exercises depicted in this story.

To Arjun, Ashvin & Anya

Rob waited for Dad to get him after school.
He waited and waited but Dad didn't come.

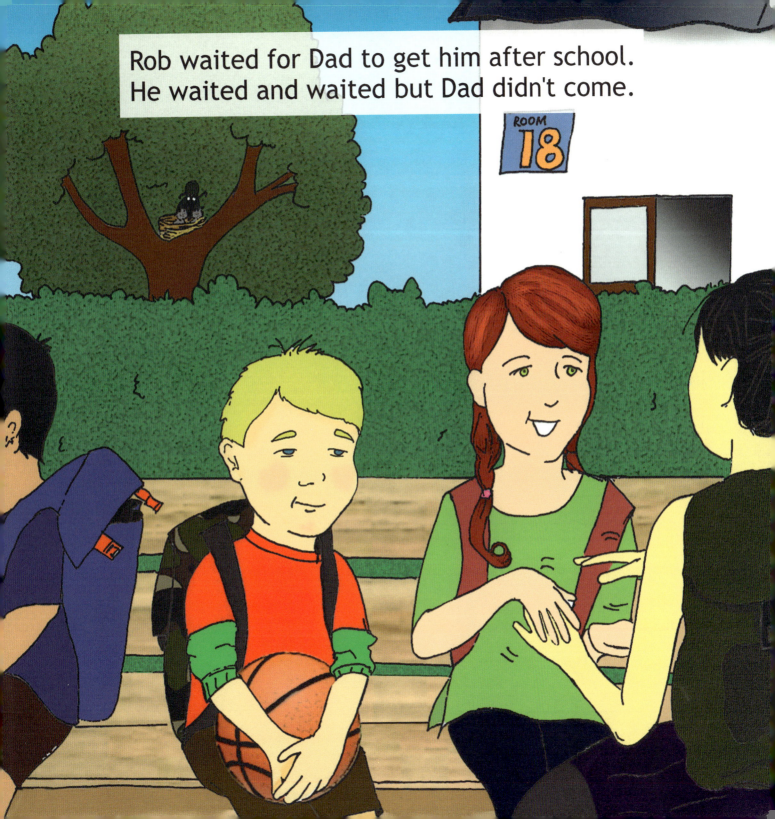

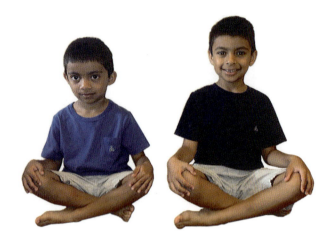

Happy or Seated Pose

Sit on the floor and cross your legs. Put your hands on your knees and sit up tall.

He waved to his friend Ravi driving home with his mum,

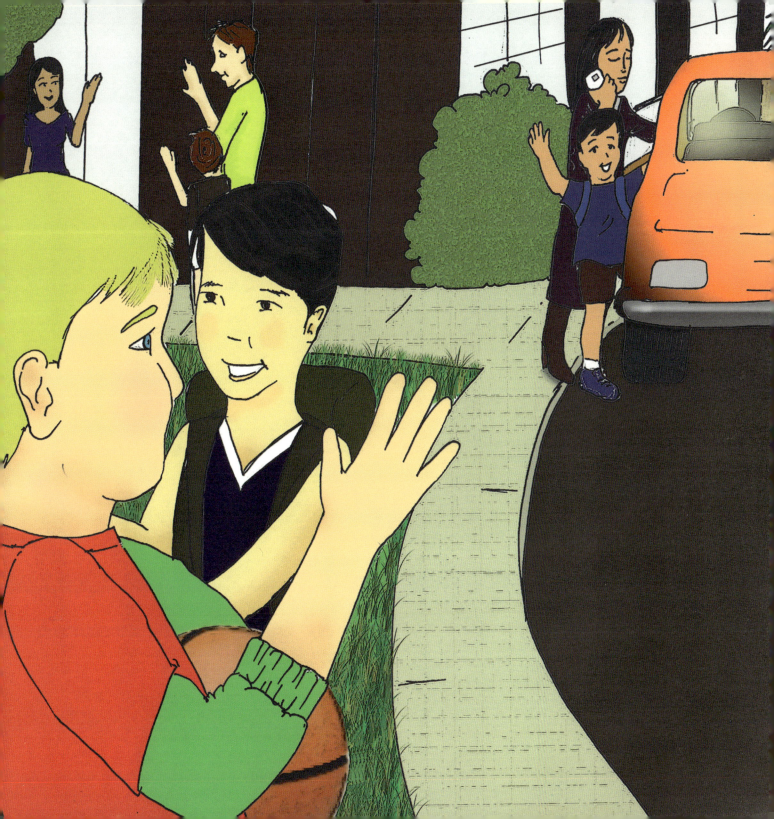

and Ally who walked home with her big brother Chad.

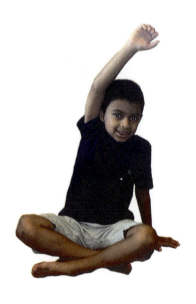

Side Stretch

Place your left hand on the floor and reach up, up, up to the ceiling with your right arm. Feel the nice stre-e-e-tch! Try it with your other arm. Make sure to wave to your friends like Rob!

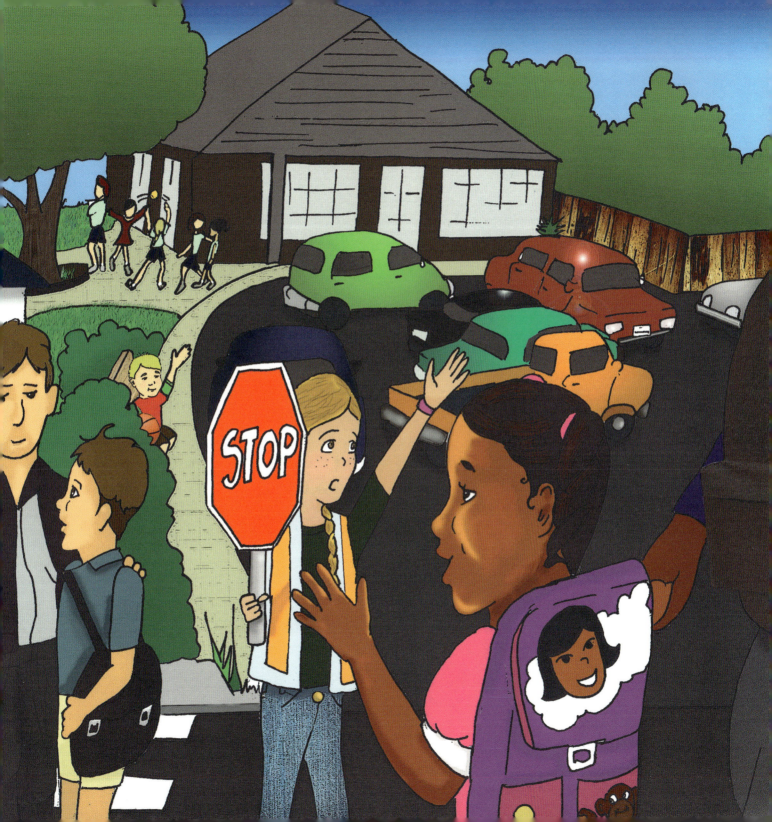

Soon the place was empty.
Still no Dad.

"What ever could have happened to Dad?" worried Rob.

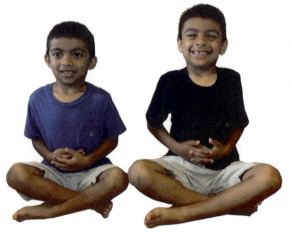

Belly Breathing

We're going to practice some deep breathing now. So make sure you've got your hands on your tummy. Breathe in through your nose and watch your tummy grow! Now breathe out and watch your tummy flatten. Try it again slowly, and again. This type of breathing makes you feel calm when you're worried.

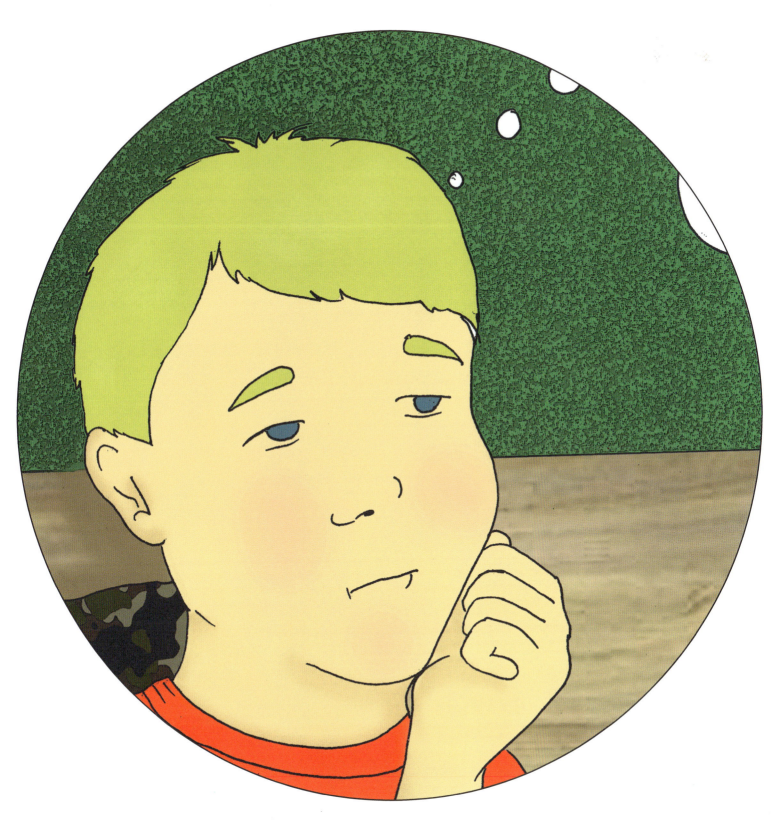

He might be fighting with pirates and forced to walk the plank.

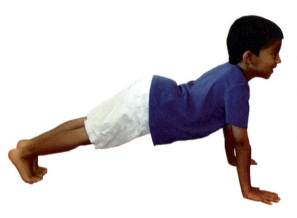

Plank Position

Kneel down and put both hands flat on the floor. Spread your fingers wide. Now put both legs out behind you. Let's see how long you can hold this position for. Let's count to ten. 1-2-3-4-5-6-7-8-10. You did it!

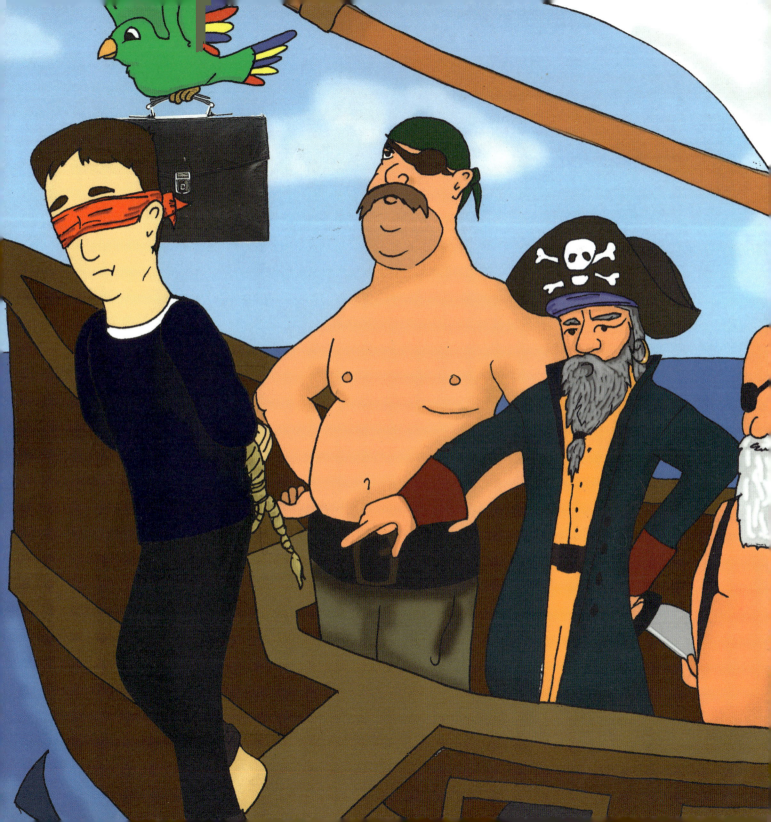

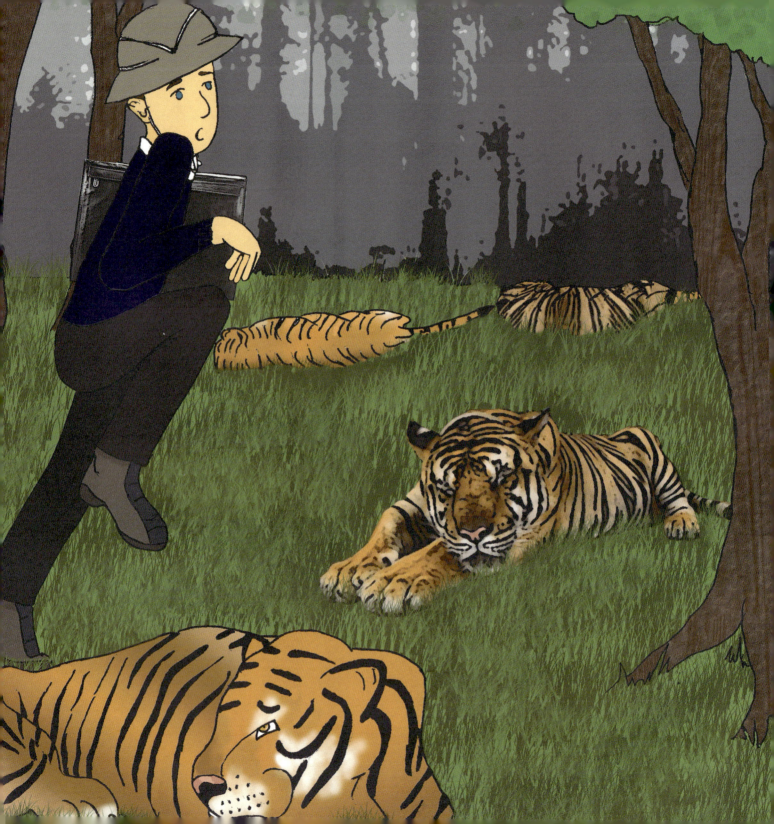

He might be tiptoeing past tigers on a lush, jungle path.

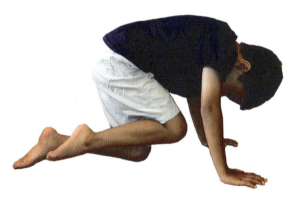

Tiger Pose

Okay, we're going to be stretching tigers now. So get back on your hands and knee and bring one knee slowly to your forehead. See if you can touch them together. Feel that stretch in your back!

Then push your knee out and arch your back. Roar like a tiger. ROAR! Do this pose using your other knee.

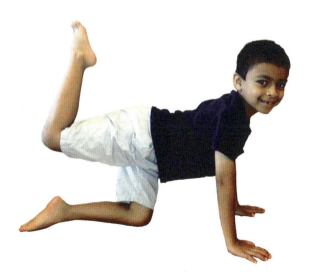

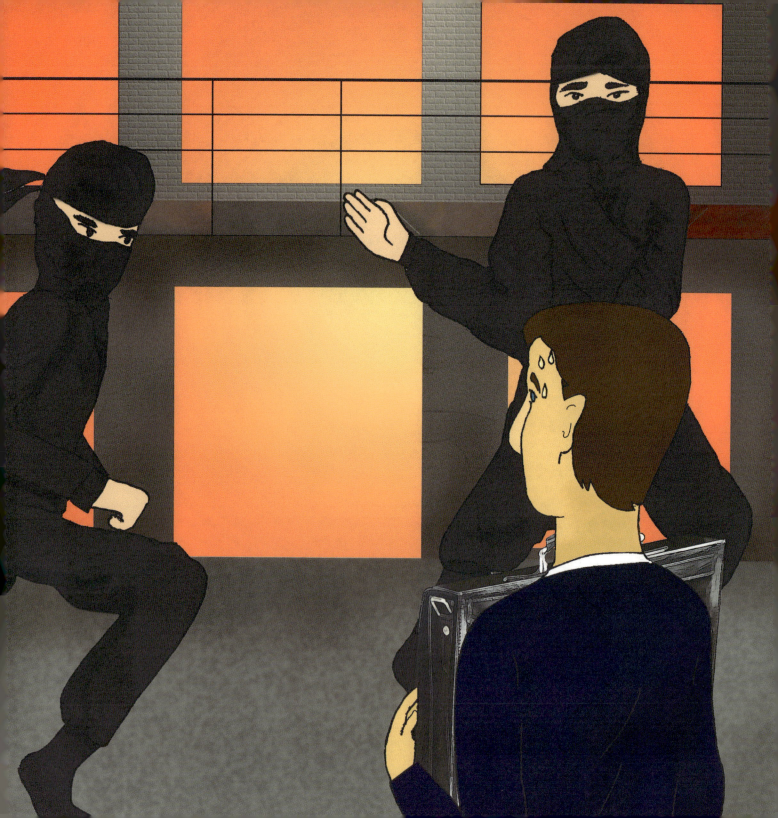

He was fighting with ninjas for defeating their master,

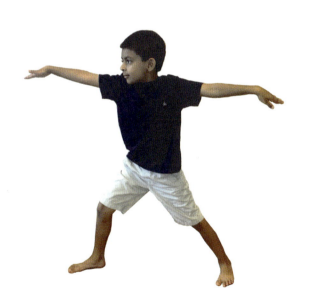

Warrior Pose Two

Yes, we are starting with number two first!
Stand tall and put your left foot backwards.
Turn your right foot so it's pointing forward
and turn the left foot slightly in.
Bend your right knee in a deep lunge. When
you feel balanced, lift your arms up to
shoulder height.
Look over your right hand.
Balance your weight in the center of the pose
and do not lean on your knee.
Remember to switch legs!

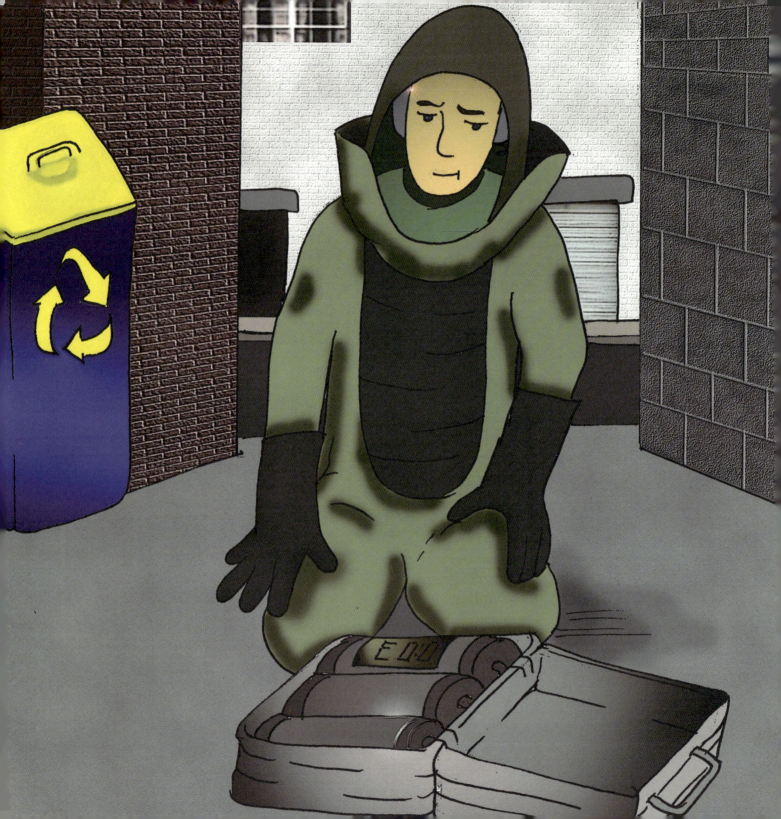

or saving the world from a bombing disaster.

Warrior Pose One

Stand tall and put your left foot backwards.
Turn your right foot so it's pointing forward
and turn the left foot slightly in.
Swing your hips to face your right foot and
lift your arms over your head.
Bend your right knee but make sure it doesn't
go over your right toe. Look up towards your
hands. Hold it for five seconds. 1,2,3,4,5!
Now switch your legs.

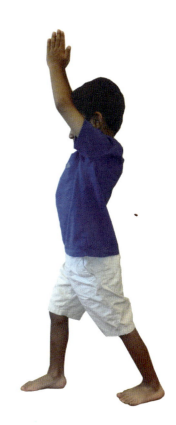

He was lost in the desert over dry, sandy dunes,

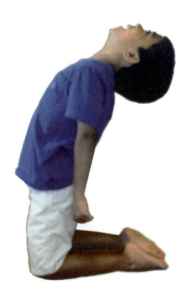

Camel Pose

We're going to pretend to be the hump on the camel. First, kneel and reach your arms back to your feet. Roll your shoulders back and push your chest towards the sky. Lean back as far as comfortable and put your head back.

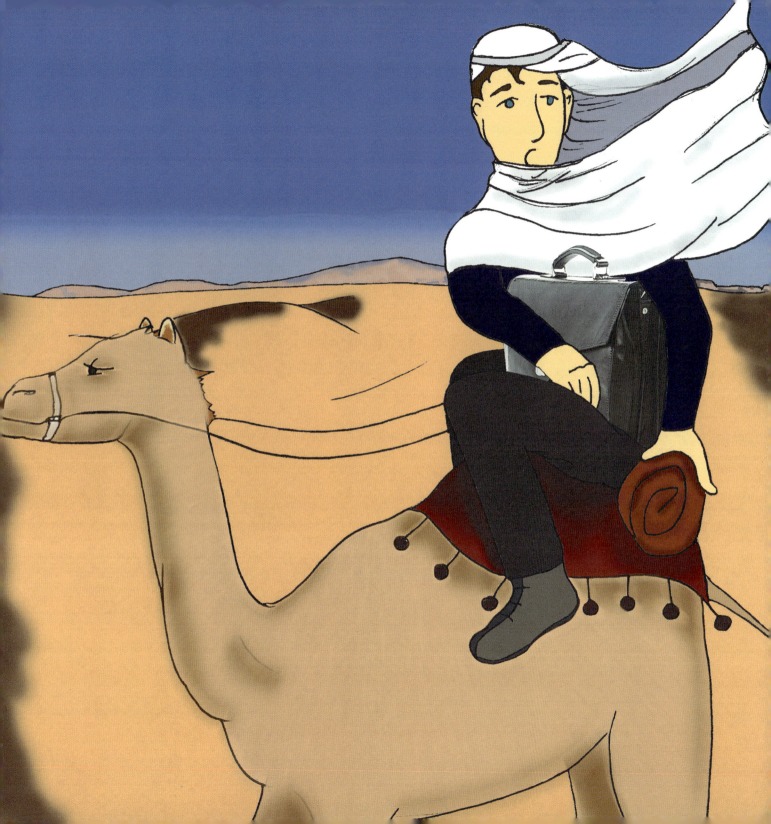

or kidnapped by aliens and sent to the moon.

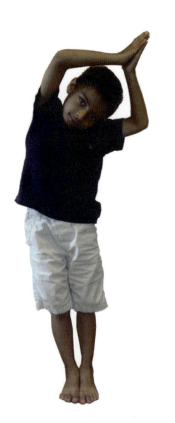

Half Moon Pose

I have taken this particular pose from Bikram Yoga.
Stand tall with your legs together.
Bring your hands up over your head.
Breathe in and then breathe out. While breathing out,
bend sideways to your left as far as you can go from
your hip sockets.
Remember to do the same thing on your right side.

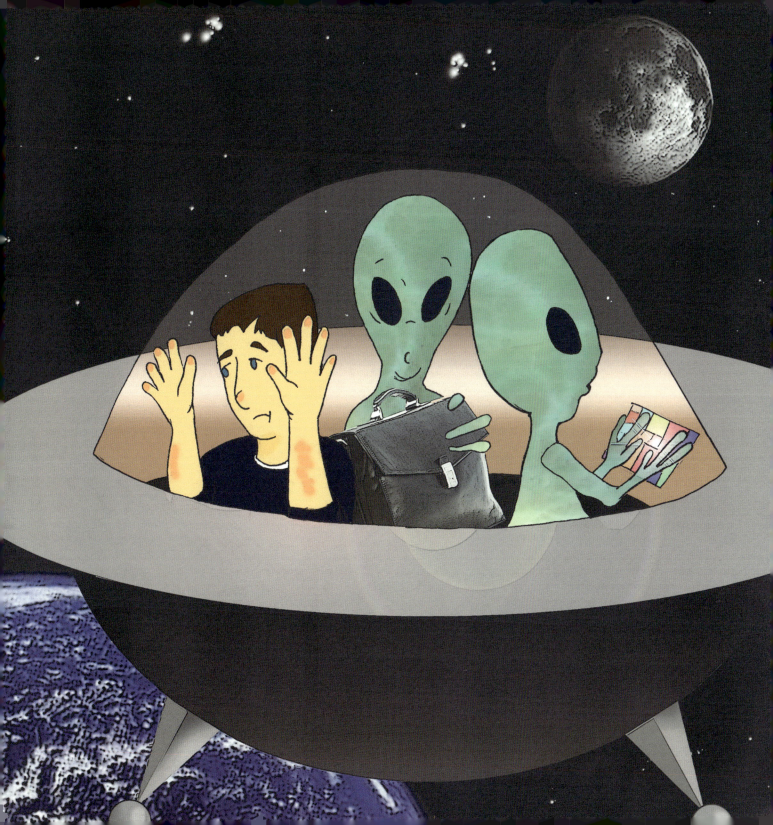

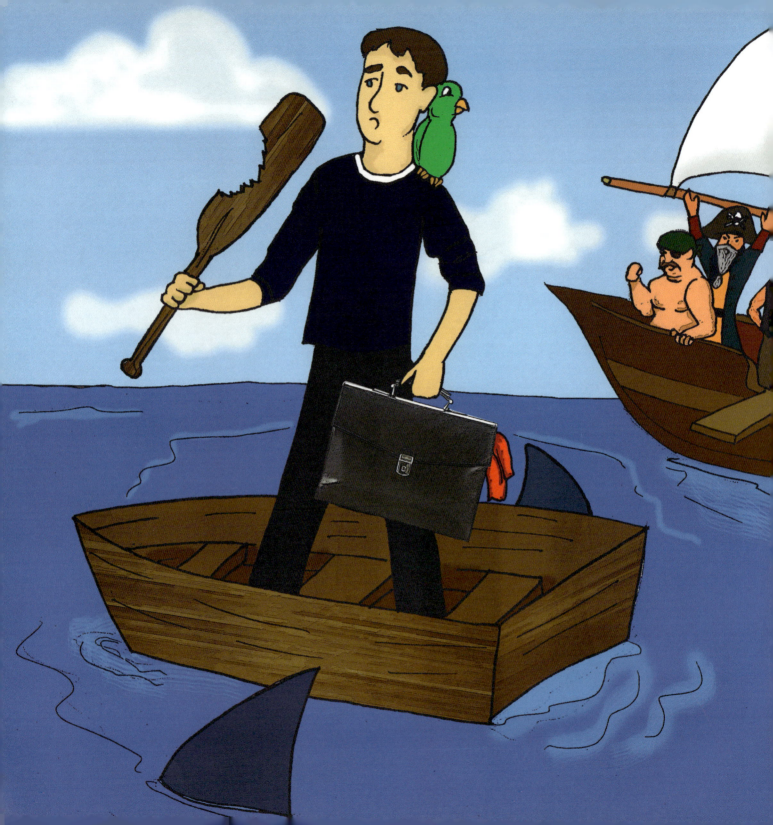

Maybe Dad was at sea and surrounded by sharks,

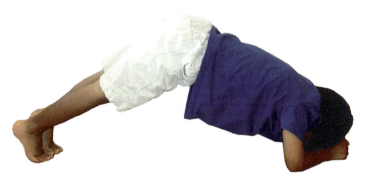

Dolphin Pose (Shark Pose)

For this pose, we're going to pretend to be shark fins. Get back on the floor on your hands and knees and make sure that your elbows all the way to your hands are pushing into the floor.

Curl your toes under your feet, then lift your knees away from the floor. Try to push your hips and butt up to the ceiling. Now you're a shark fin!

or monsters have chained him to a cave in the dark.

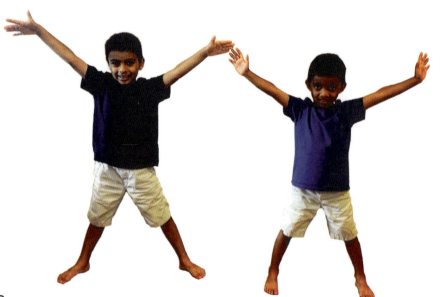

Star Pose

Oh no! You've been chained to the cave like Rob's dad!

Stand with your legs apart and your arms out straight and to your sides, so you look like a star.

Try to break free from the chains...

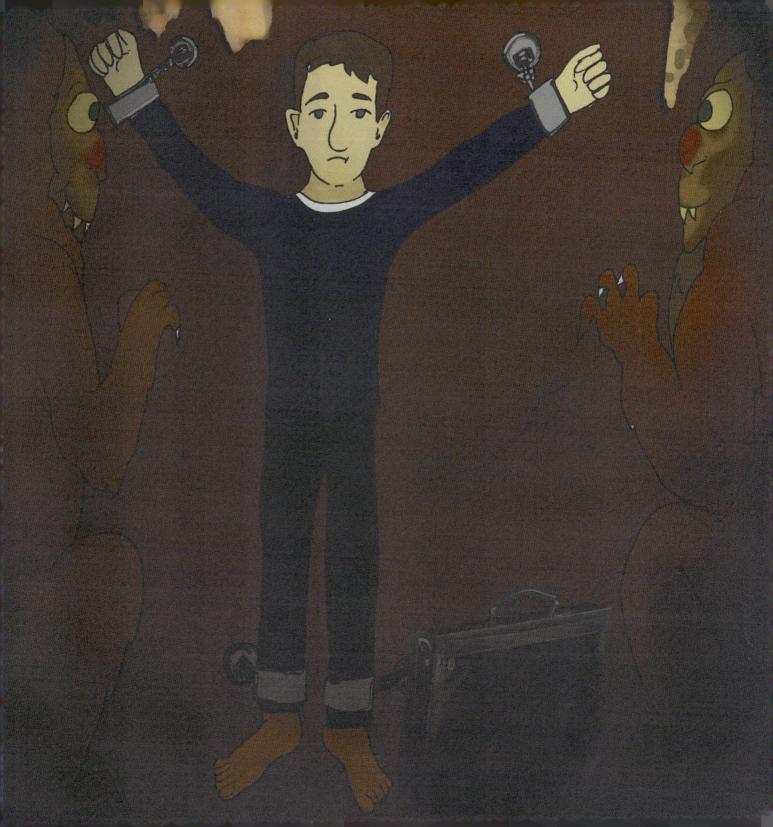

"Poor Dad," thought Rob, "what will he ever do?"
Just then, round the corner, came Mrs. Lu.
"Well then, Rob," she said, "looks like someone's
forgotten you.

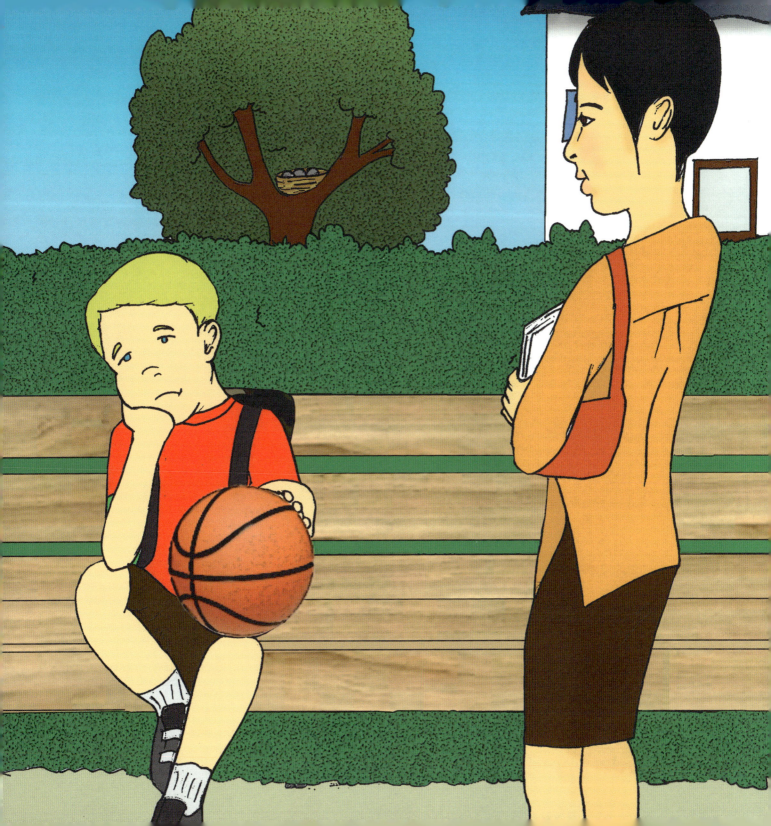

Let's go to the office. We'll call home for you too."

Then, speeding down the road came Dad in his jeep.
He scrambled out the car and got to his feet.

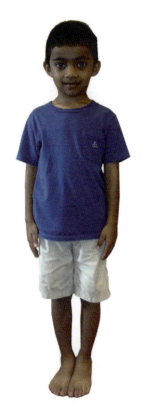

Tadasana or Mountain Pose

Stand tall with your feet apart and your toes facing forward.
Hands at your sides. Think of a string attached to the top of
your head pulling it up toward the sky. Feel the heels of
your feet planted firmly on the ground.

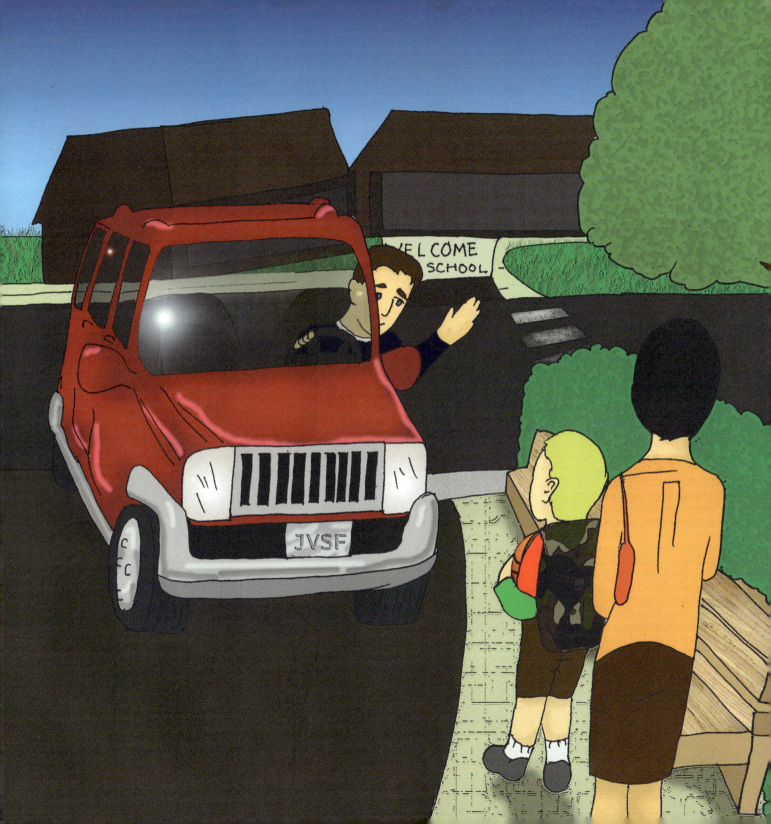

He said he was at a meeting that ran really late.
And even Rob believed him until he saw
Dad's black briefcase.

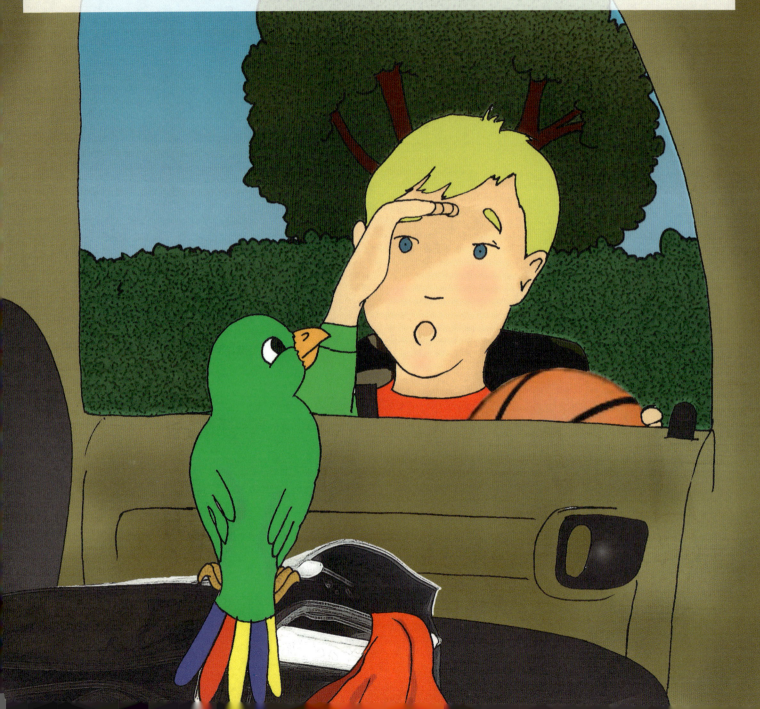

Made in the USA
Charleston, SC
21 September 2013